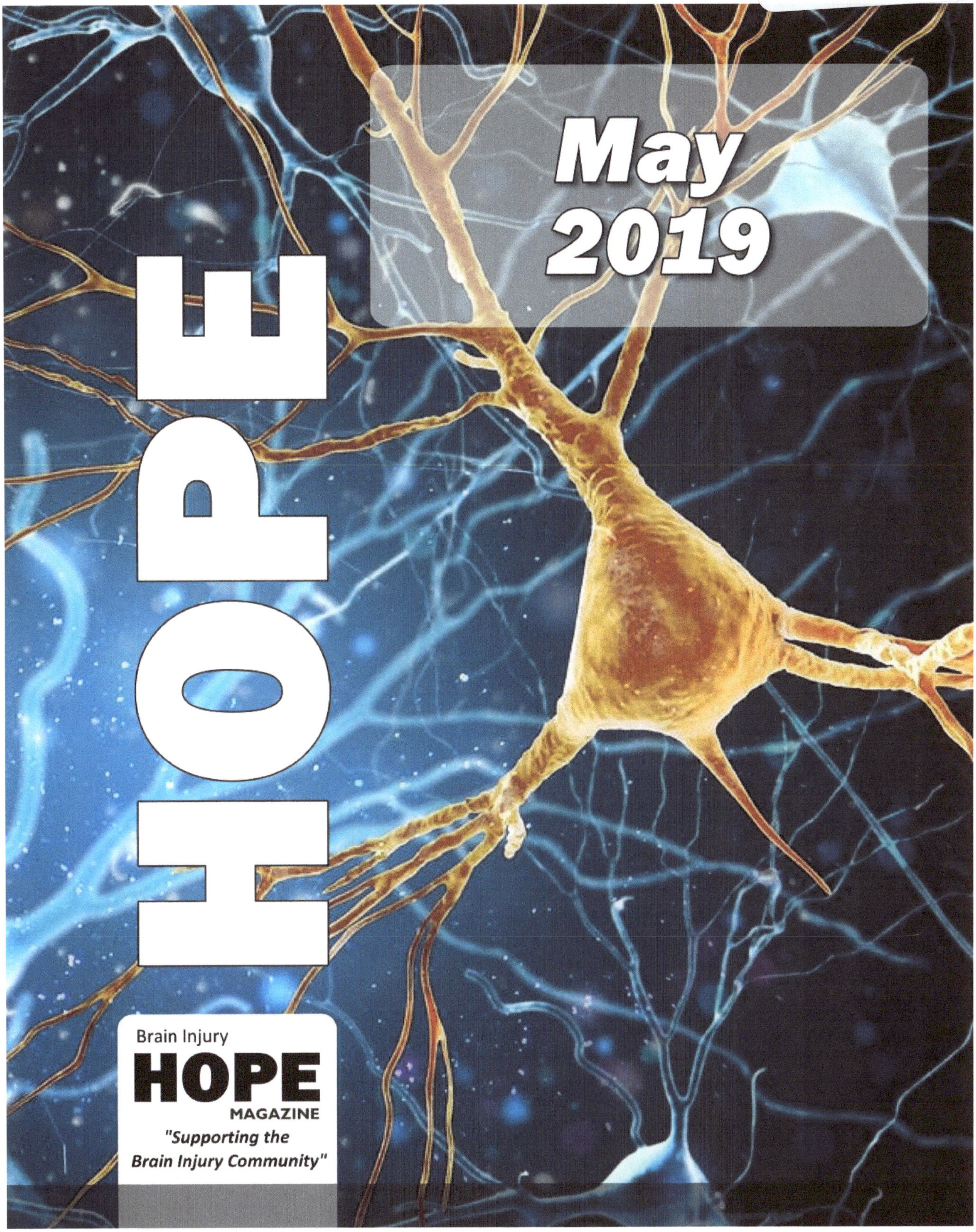

May
2019

HOPE

Brain Injury
HOPE
MAGAZINE
*"Supporting the
Brain Injury Community"*

Welcome

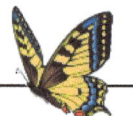

HOPE MAGAZINE

Serving the Brain Injury Community

May 2019

Publisher
David A. Grant

Editor
Sarah Grant

Our Contributors

Nicole Bingaman
Patrick Brigham
Jennifer Collins
Debra Gorman
Rhonda Johnson
Ric Johnson
Norma Myers
Laurie Oleksa
Shannon Sharman

Welcome to the May 2019 issue of HOPE Magazine

Brain injury is unlike most other injuries. While the survivor seems to often be the attention of focus, there are countless others who are profoundly affected.

From parents to children, to spouses and friends, each one carries the weight of life after brain injury.

In this month's issue, we feature several stories from caregivers, spouses, and family members of brain injury survivors. I can speak from immensely personal experience when I share that my wife Sarah had it tougher than I did during the time following my injury.

While I have forgotten most of 2011, she remembers it in painful detail.

To those who have shown superhuman courage in sharing their stories this month, I thank you. Your words will help countless others around the world.

Peace,

David A. Grant
Publisher

Contents

What's Inside

May 2019

"Count your age by friends, not years. Count your life by smiles, not tears."

-John Lennon

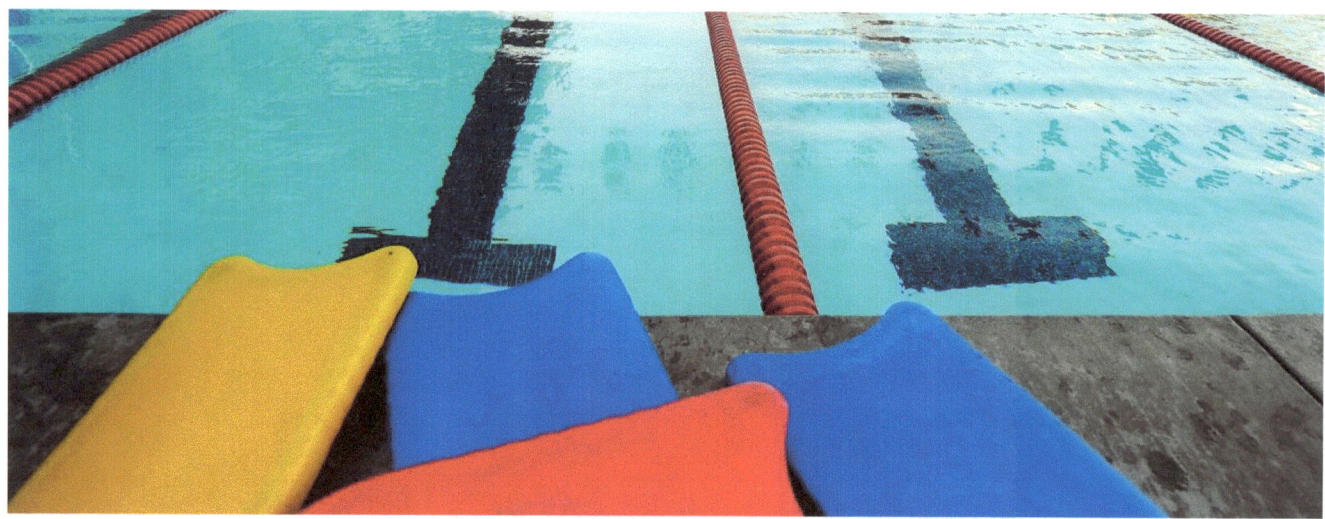

Danny's Journey

By Laurie Oleksa

Our story began in June of 2003. My son Danny was ten days away from his twelfth birthday when he suffered a severe anoxic brain injury. At the time, he was a bright, athletic, social kid with a great sense of humor.

I left Danny in our car while I ran into our public library for a couple of minutes. When I returned to the car, Danny was on the grass outside our car and a man (who, ironically, is a friend of ours) was performing CPR. A woman had come out to her car and found Danny with the seatbelt wrapped around his neck and he was hanging outside the vehicle. Unfortunately, no one witnessed what happened so we have no idea, but suspect someone might have tried to steal the car without realizing he was in it.

> "A woman had come out to her car and found Danny with the seatbelt wrapped around his neck and he was hanging outside the vehicle."

What we have quickly learned is that an anoxic brain injury can be more devastating than a blunt traumatic brain injury because of the global damage that occurs. During the more than seven months he spent in Mary Free Bed Rehabilitation Hospital, we watched patient after patient come in with severe trauma to a portion of their brain, yet they walked out with minimal damage compared to Danny, despite the fact that he didn't suffer even a scratch to his head. He did obviously suffer severe bruising to the neck, but those bruises faded long before the reality of his injury set in.

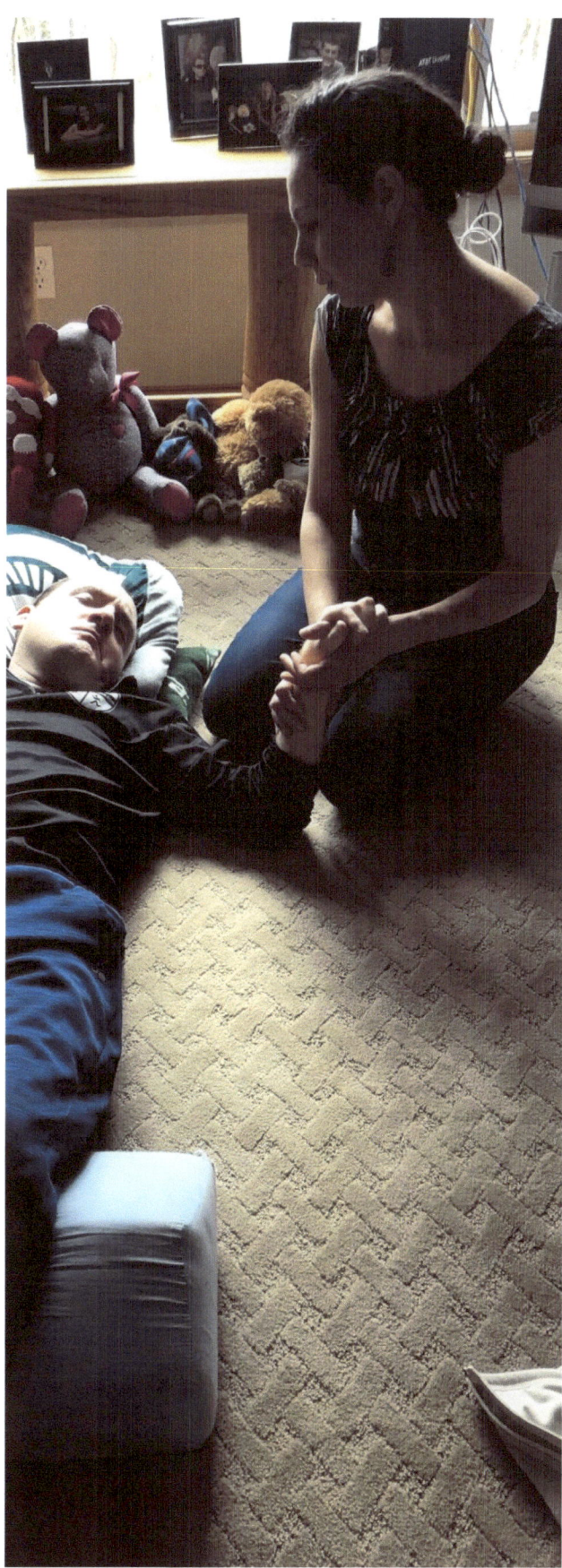

His brain injury has left him non-verbal, bound to a wheelchair due to a lack of any functional movement, tube fed and cortically visually impaired. He also has a seizure disorder and while most of his seizures are relatively mild, he does require oxygen following some of his harder episodes due to a drop in his oxygen level.

Our journey has been full of tears and heartbreak, but also much joy and new relationships. Danny played soccer, baseball and golf, but his passion was for ice hockey. Following in his older sister Caitlin's footsteps, he began playing hockey when he was four years old. At the time of his injury he was playing his fourth year of travel hockey.

Because of the great amount of time spent with his hockey team, his best friends were mainly his teammates. Following the injury, those friendships faded away with time, especially due to their young age, a lack of that common activity level and Danny's inability to communicate with his friends. The loss of a social circle has been one of the most difficult aspects of our situation. Social media is a wonderful way to stay connected, but also serves as a source of heartbreak as I have seen his friends go to Proms, graduate from high school and college, get married and have babies.

But we are fortunate to have my three closest friends and their families that have stayed a strong source of love and support for Danny, Caitlin and myself. This became especially important to me when Danny's dad left our marriage four years after the accident however, I'm grateful that he has stayed a loving, involved father to Danny and Caitlin. We are blessed beyond measure by these friendships.

I do want to share a part of Danny's recovery that has been so exciting. In August of 2017, I hired Miranda, a recreation therapist, to do aquatic therapy with Danny because he was aging out of school and was not going to have access to the pool anymore. As I stated earlier, he has no functional movement so up until then, the time he spent in the pool at his school was an opportunity to just relax and have his range of motion worked on to prevent further contractures. That is what I expected Miranda to continue to do with Danny.

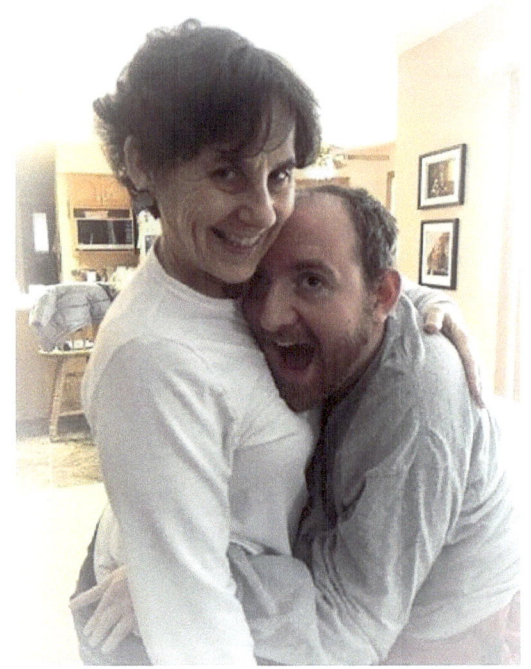

After a couple months of working with Danny in the pool, Miranda began to do exercises with him requesting him to follow commands through body movements. He responded to these commands immediately. He also showed memory of the exercises from session to session by starting to do them before Miranda would give him commands. His ability to process her verbal commands and then to follow the commands with intentional body movements is so impressive.

Danny is now able to lower his legs all the way down until his bottom is against the side of the pool. He can then raise and lower them on command. Today he even followed her directions to move his legs to the right and to the left. I am truly amazed by his ability to do this immediately. We have known that Danny was alert and aware of his surroundings by his positive responses to people he knows (even to his friends who only come around once or twice a year) and his laughter at jokes and funny situations. But I never imagined he could process and then follow through with commands requiring functional movements.

This all happened fourteen years post-accident. So never let anyone tell you there will be no more progress, like we were told after one year post-accident. Danny has not been able to replicate these skills out of the water yet, but the fact that he is aware that we now know what he is capable of has given him confidence and a sense of pride. Every single day I am amazed by Danny's patience and tolerance of the many challenges he faces. To go from being social and active to completely reliant on others for all of your basic needs and to having extremely limited communication skills has to be incredibly frustrating. Yet, he seems very content and at peace with what life has dealt him. My heart swells with pride for the young man he has become.

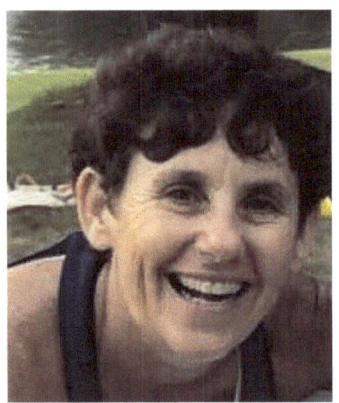

Meet Laurie Oleksa

Laurie writes…

" I am a retired teacher and spent all 33 years of my teaching career working with students with special needs at a developmental center in Battle Creek, MI. Following Danny's accident, he became a student at that same school, so I was able to be very involved in his education. I now spend my days working part time at our local YMCA, where Danny is also a member. In August 2019 I will be competing in my 2nd Half Ironman event in Traverse City, MI."

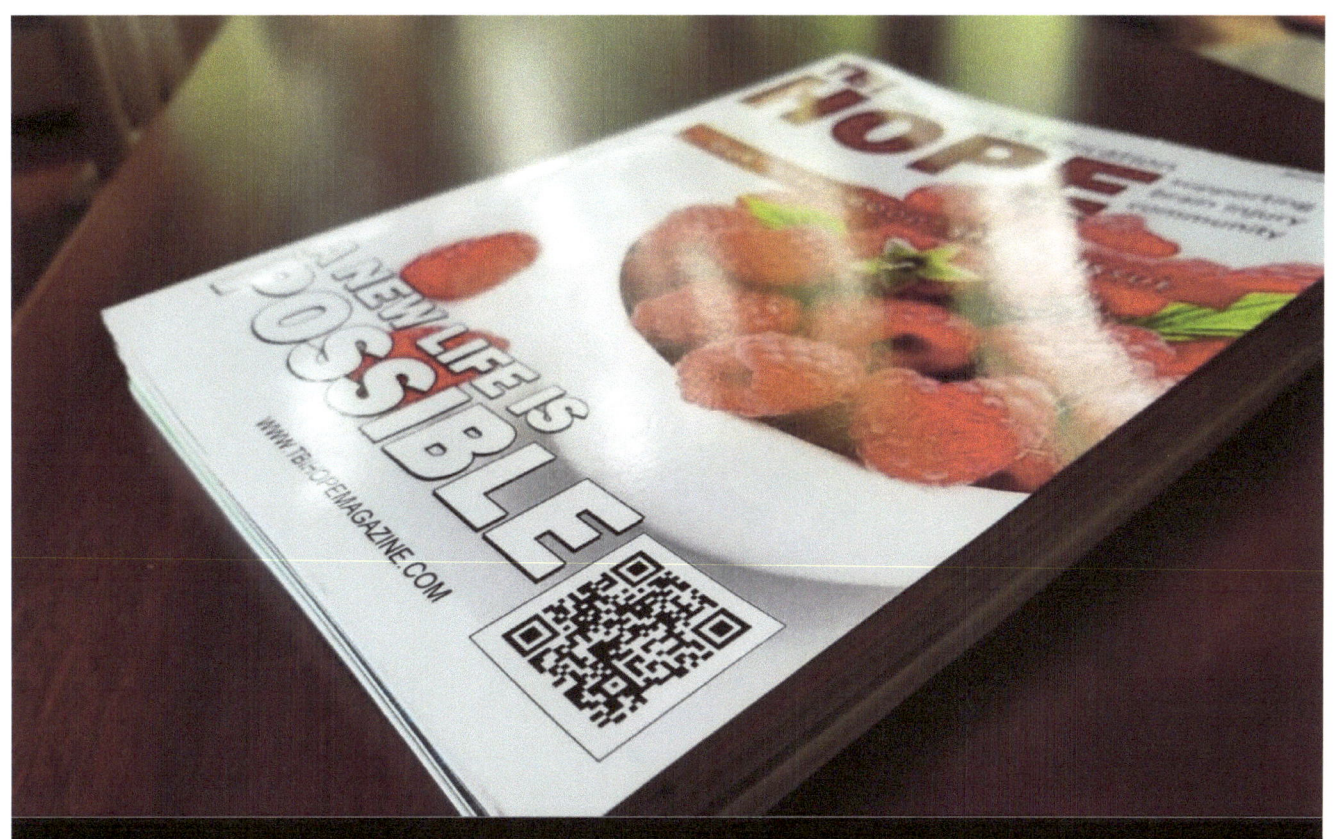

HOPE MAGAZINE

Caregiver Stories Wanted!

We are looking for stories from a caregiver's perspective for HOPE Magazine. Your experience has worth and value - and can help others affected by brain injury.

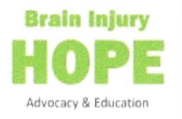

Brain Injury
HOPE
Advocacy & Education

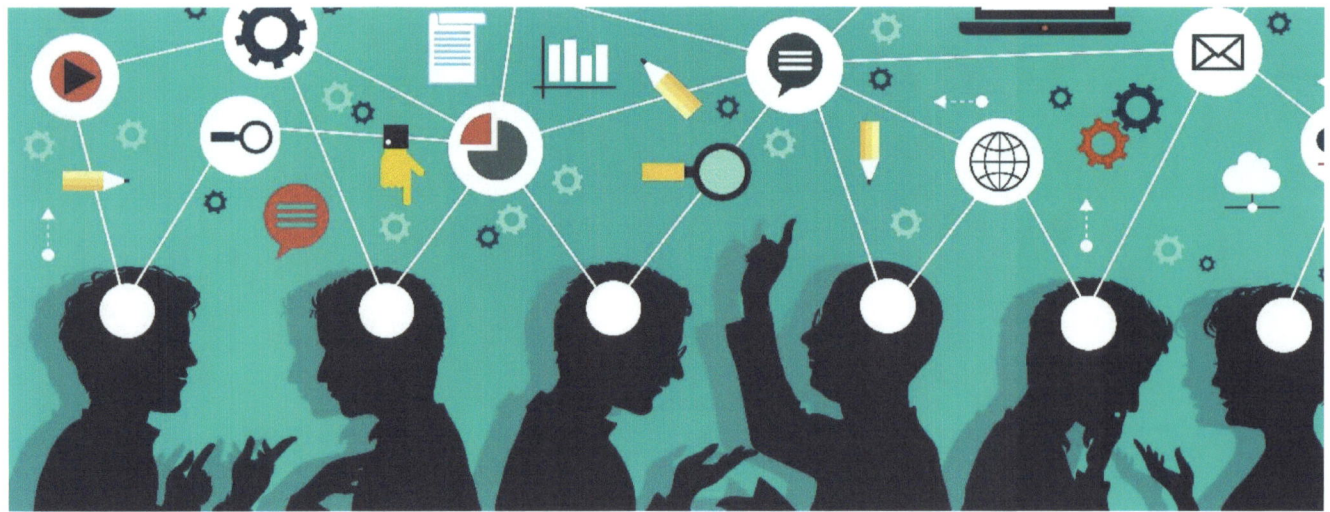

The Healing Power of Sharing
By Ric Johnson

"Heard you had a traumatic brain injury. You look great. What the heck does that mean? Sorry, don't have time to hang around. See ya later."

Seems that is how many friends and other people react when we are meeting up with them. It could be the first time or the tenth time, most people do not understand there is a huge difference between "broke my brain" and "broke my arm."

For our families, it is a little better, since they are living through the injury as well. But for non-survivors, trying to understand us is the same as trying to smell the color nine. Last March was Brain Injury Awareness Month but survivors should make every month a brain injury awareness month. So how do I, or you, make people more aware and understanding about brain injury?

> "Last March was Brain Injury Awareness Month but survivors should make every month a brain injury awareness month."

Here are the steps I use:

1) A two-to-three minute story about my injury.
2) A two-minute story about the therapies I went through.
3) Yes, my injury happened fifteen years ago, but I am still recovering. In fact, recovery means my brain is actually still re-wiring itself.

4) Explain how much energy I need to do anything, whether it is physical or mental, and that it's harder than anything I have done before.
5) What my brain (and I) heard or saw and that processing that information is slower than before. It takes more time to process.
6) If I did not have a good night's sleep, the next day may be a less than a productive day.
7) If I say I cannot do something, I am not faking it. Every day is a different day. I could do this yesterday, but not today, or vice versa.
8) Did I repeat myself? Sorry, but short-term memory comes and goes.
9) If I don't seem to be talking very well it's because I have aphasia, which means saying the "wrong" word is a fact of my life. It is all about language skills.

Those nine steps take about ten minutes. Most people seem to get distracted after ten minutes. Unlike survivors, non-survivors have a fast-paced life, especially if they have kids in tow. I also think that being able to talk to others about myself is a piece of my "sense-of-self."

It seems that the more I tell my story, the better I understand myself.

> ## "It seems that the more I tell my story, the better I understand myself."

Those nine steps take about ten minutes. Most people seem to get distracted after ten minutes. Unlike survivors, non-survivors have a fast-paced life, especially if they have kids in tow. I also think that being able to talk to others about myself is a piece of my "sense-of-self." Seems that the more I tell my story, the better I understand myself.

During the first few years, I tried not to look in the mirror. If I did, I only saw my scars and a blank look in my eyes. Looking at the mirror now, I see me, older with grayer hair but really me. I am able to smile at my reflection and say "way to go, look at all we (the royal we) have gone through." It helps me think that I will be able to handle pretty much anything that could happen today or in future days. Recovery never stops as long as I stop grieving about my past; sense-of-self keeps me moving toward the future.

Telling my story to other people is also the same story-telling that I do during the local support group I attend every month. During those meetings, I tell my tips or techniques that are helping me and hopefully will help other members of the group, and I listen to their tips. Talking to "non-family or friends" is really helping them know that after a brain injury a survivor's life is at a crossroads. For many of us, there are no physical cues. The "mental" cues are mostly unseen. For the general public, fatigue can look like we are milking our injury or trying to get sympathy. After fifteen years, I have never seen a survivor asking for sympathy. If I am asking for help there is a reason and since others can't see my brain I need to tell them what is going on. Sometimes asking for help is daunting. But there is no shame.

For me, working in the same company for over thirty-eight years in the same department and in the same "job" for over four years, asking for help is hard. Because of my short-term memory troubles, I write many notes and post them all over my desk. Many times a task will come up, not a task I do daily, but frequently, and at that particular time, I have no idea what I need to do. When that happens, I need to find the "correct" note to use to work on that task.

> "If I am asking for help there is a reason and since others can't see my brain I need to tell them what is going on."

If I can't find the note, or if the process to finish the task has changed, I will definitely need to have somebody walk me through the task and let me re-write my note before they leave. I may even ask them to proofread my note or have me read it back. I need to remind my co-workers that short-term memory is not a "senior moment," for me, it's a daily moment.

Many times in this article I have used the word I or me, but using "we" instead probably would not have changed the text I wrote. Tell your story. Let people know about you and your injury. It gets easier each time you tell it.

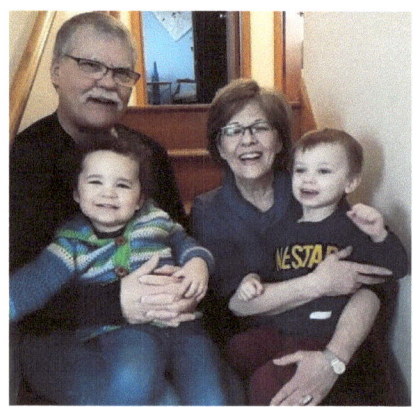

Meet Ric Johnson

Ric Johnson is a husband, father, and grandfather. A survivor from a traumatic brain injury of 15+ years. Ric is also a member of the Speaker Bureau for the Minnesota Brain Injury Alliance, and facilitator for The Courage Kenny Brain Injury Support Group.

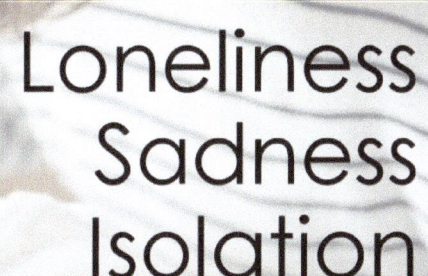

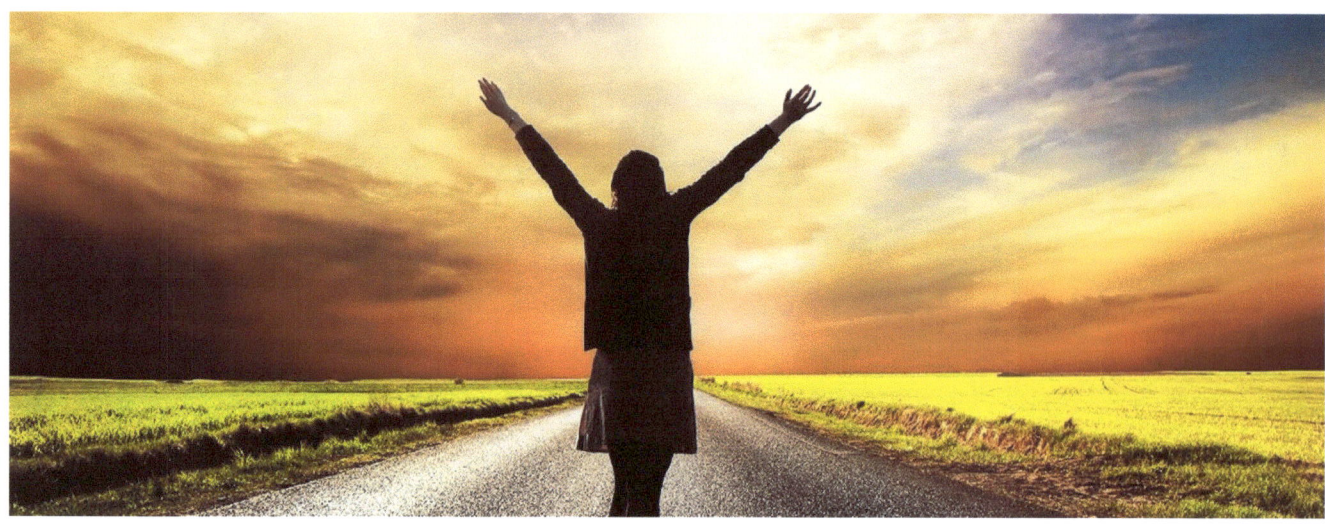

Loving the New Me

By Shannon Sharman

I have contributed twice to this magazine. Once straight out of hospital and once two years later. Like everyone else, life has gotten busy and I have not had much time to reflect over the past five years post acquired brain injury. I wanted to talk about the things I was told I'd never do because I was not defined by my brain injury. It's a funny thing hearing people say they were told they would never and could never do certain things.

> "I wanted to talk about the things I was told I'd never do because I was not defined by my brain injury."

Yes, sometimes 'they' get it right, sometimes life does stop, and you don't get a chance to be the person you wanted to be. However, I am seeing time and time again these miraculous people who use what they have learnt through brain injury to educate and help countless other survivors and their families. I know I wouldn't be the same without my brain injury family and Queensland's STEPS (Skills to Enable People and Places) program.

I was a driven, hard-working person studying a Bachelor of Communications whilst working full time in a busy Queensland hospital. I won't go through my lengthy four-month hospital stay at the place where I aspire to work: Princess Alexandra Hospital. I will give you a quick summary (you can always look me up in December 2015's issue of Hope & Inspiration), I had three hemorrhages and growth from a benign tumour of the midbrain part of the brainstem (the tumour named Cavernous Haemangioma).

I went through five brain surgeries due to hospital-acquired infections and inserting a VP shunt for hydrocephalus. I worked aimlessly to learn to walk, talk, and eat again. I worked hard, but do not miss

"If I wasn't such a stubborn person, I may have given up several times throughout the last five years. Yes, I even mean as recently as six weeks ago."

this. I would not be alive without my family always being there and never giving up on me. Family is a powerful thing. I also believe heavily that my Neurosurgeon is god (Dr Sarah Olson). I mean, brainstem surgery is not a procedure done often in Australia and certainly not a survival one, but magic was involved on that day Friday 16th, May 2014.

If I wasn't such a stubborn person, I may have given up several times throughout the last five years. Yes, I even mean as recently as six weeks ago. I had an exacerbation of my neurological symptoms that I encountered when I had my first brain hemorrhage in 2014, suffice to say my family made me go back to hospital. Here I was diagnosed as having partial seizures.

I was told I could not drive or work till I was able to see a Neurologist. I was put on a brutal medicine that made it impossible to fall pregnant (I am in my child-bearing years). I did not agree with this diagnosis and I fell into a well of despair as once again I was going through trying to regain my job and license.

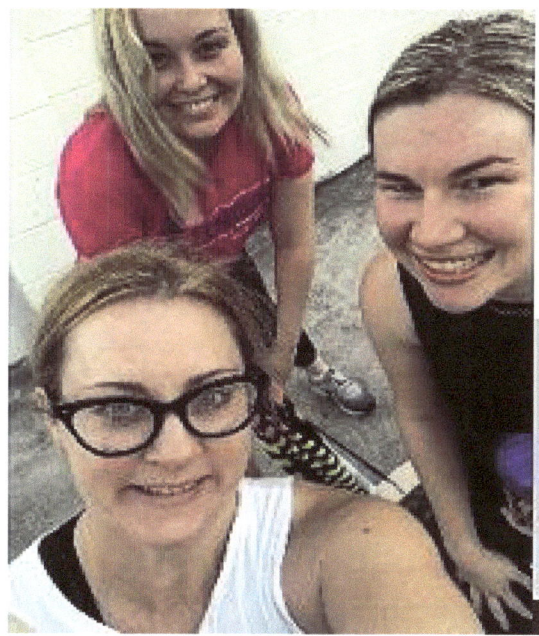

I've just recently had the diagnosis reversed as it was incorrect and therefore, I can drive and work again. I do not hold anyone responsible for this as they thought they saw something that was not there and was diagnosing as per their education. Whenever something like this happens, I get a little madder at life however, this will not throw me off track. I have a goal. This goal is my mission and I fully believe the reason I survived the incredible.

When I was in hospital, I fell in love with medicine. I envied the nurses who were able to assist the newly brain-injured people. Some nurses made me cringe at how bad they were with me. I mean, why get into nursing with acquired brain injury if you are unable to understand and care for the ups and downs that come with acquired brain injury! But, believe me, I had some real compassionate souls look after me (some a little too sad for me, one used to cry whenever she saw me so I thought I was dying). That was it, I found that one thing most people spend their whole life looking for, my dream, my purpose. I had a long way to go, my aim was to become a nurse.

I spent the last three years pushing myself to learn to live without fear, learn to drive with an eyepatch and study a Diploma of Nursing and work as a graduate nurse helping others. But recently, I have needed more, and I am not helping as much as I hoped. I strive to learn. I now aim to be a Nurse Practitioner (a high-level nurse) who specializes in Brain Tumors (benign and cancerous). I have two more years until I am a Registered Nurse with a Bachelor of Nursing. I spend every spare minute studying. I must be the best; I have a lot to prove. Therefore, watch this space, because one day you'll see me speaking at conferences about this very story!

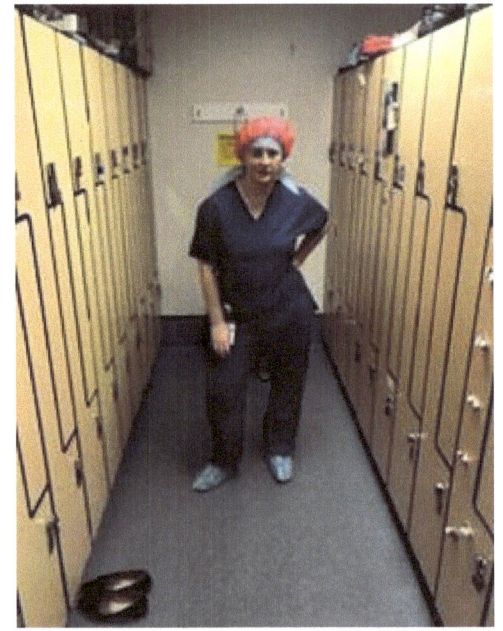

Meet Shannon Sharman

Shannon was born in Perth, Western Australia and now lives in Brisbane, Australia. Shannon married her fiancé of eight years.

She has a real passion for acting and loves going to the movies. Shannon is currently enrolled at the Queensland University of Technology and has a true passion to help others through charity work and is a volunteer at the hospital that saved her life.

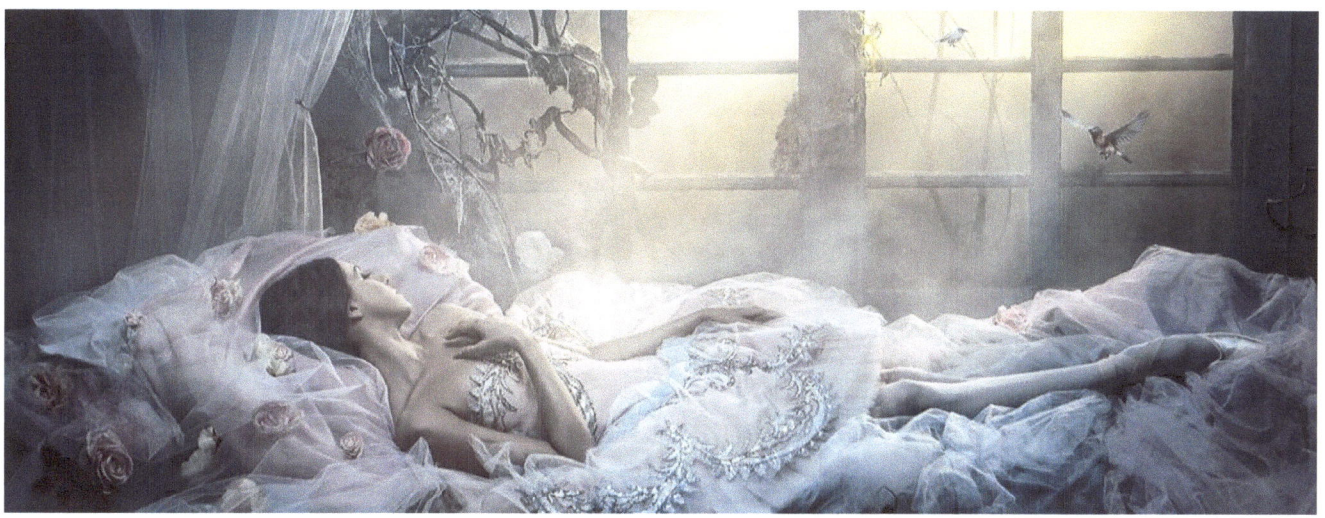

Sleeping Beauty
By Jennifer Collins

Not everyone can recall the exact moment they learned just how cruel the world can be. I still remember the day my parents came home from my sister's track meet. They should have been happy. They should have been proud of their oldest daughter for her determination and will to even step foot on the track; for the average person cringes at the mere idea of running timed laps around a hopeless ring of asphalt. But, instead, they were left visibly shaken. My family has always been anything but normal.

On March 28th, 1997, my older sister Joan was hit by a car. Upon impact she was thrown fifty feet, landing on her head. Ultimately airlifted to the Children's Hospital of Philadelphia, my parents spent a harrowing month waiting for their straight "A" third-grade daughter to awaken from her coma. My parents were swiftly told to say their last goodbyes to their eight year old daughter, because even if she did somehow survive, she would be deemed a "vegetable."

> "While other kids her age were going to school and playing with their friends, Joan was struggling to learn her own name."

But my sister was strong, and she knew how to fight. For the next few months, Joan spent her days learning how to walk and talk again. While other kids her age were going to school and playing with their friends, Joan was struggling to learn her own name. My sister seemed to defy the odds when she successfully learned how to walk, talk, and do so with ease. She even earned herself the nickname "sleeping beauty" by doctors and nurses, because after the accident, her hair was caked with vomit and twigs, but her face was left with just a small scratch. While she still struggled with severe mental setbacks, the doctors approached my parents stating that they have "never seen anything like this before," and that my parents must have connections with "the man upstairs."

Although my parents knew the Joan that existed before her accident, I never knew my sister as being any other way. I was born just a few years later, on August 28, 1999. At a young age, I had to grow up and become an adult, a mentor, for my older sister. I prompted Joan not to eat with her fingers, helped her to put on a matching outfit, and constantly reminded her to brush her teeth and shower.

There was little time for the transition from my childhood into adulthood, as I not only had to take care of myself, but another human being as well. One of my earliest memories is of the time my parents decided to let her try community college. Just a few days into her first week I remember holding onto my mother's hand as she dragged me around the campus, frantically searching for my lost and confused older sister.

Although I was young at the time, I can still remember the panic in my mother's eyes. I quickly became accustomed to being on the hunt for Joan. To this day, a trip to the mall can never be accomplished without searching for my sister. Even when equipped with a cell phone, she never seems to be able to find the phone, turn it on, or even answer it.

Whether she's screaming out the lyrics to a song in the middle of the supermarket or forgetting to put clothes on and coming out

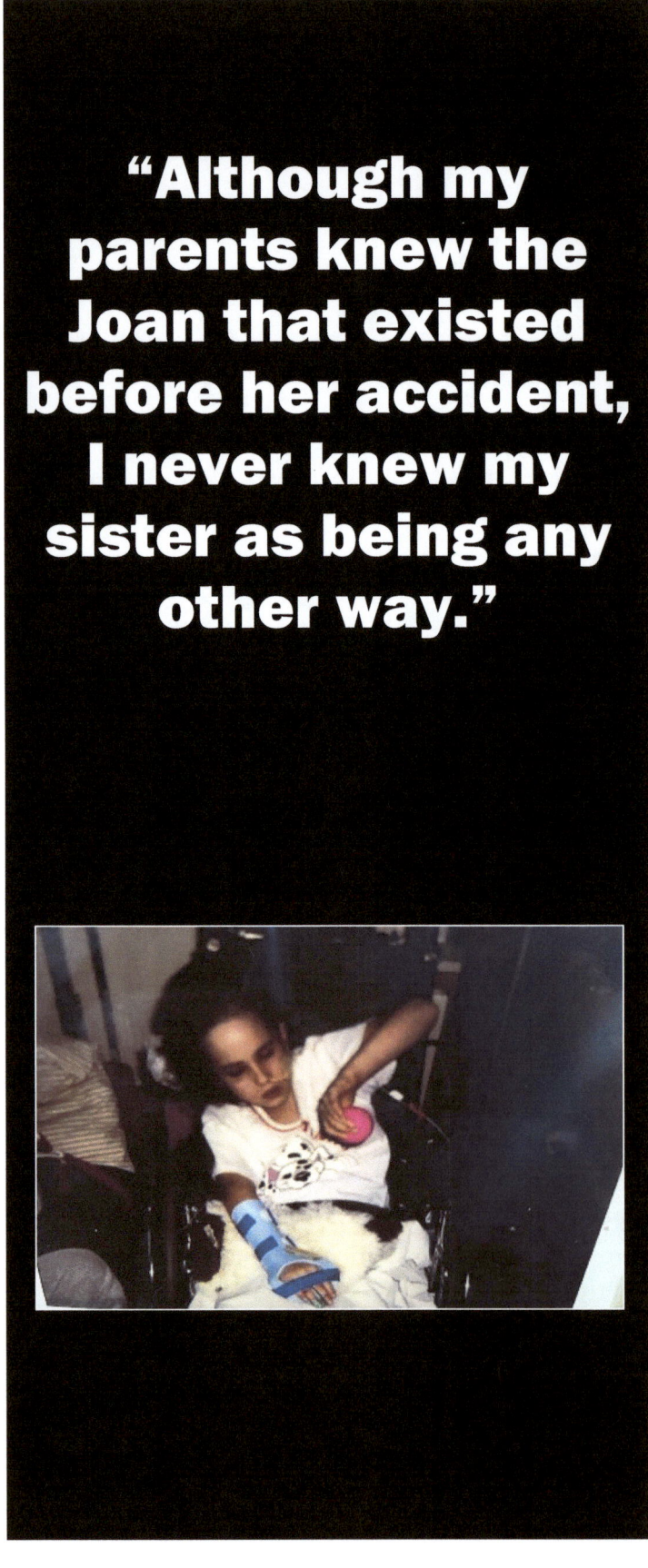

"Although my parents knew the Joan that existed before her accident, I never knew my sister as being any other way."

of our house naked, having a sister like Joan can be extremely frustrating and embarrassing.

More importantly though, growing up with Joan has taught me so many lessons that I may have never learned without her. I remember one day when my parents came home from one of Joan's track meets. They were visibly shaken. I later found out that Joan's track teammates helped her to put her leotard on backwards, as some kind of joke.

I learned the harsh lesson of just how cruel people can be. Joan, unable to comprehend the full extent of the situation, continued to smile. My sister has taught me to stay humble, and value absolutely everything that I have, because it can all be taken away within seconds. Most importantly, she has taught me to be resilient, to try new things, and to push myself beyond the boundaries that others have set for me.

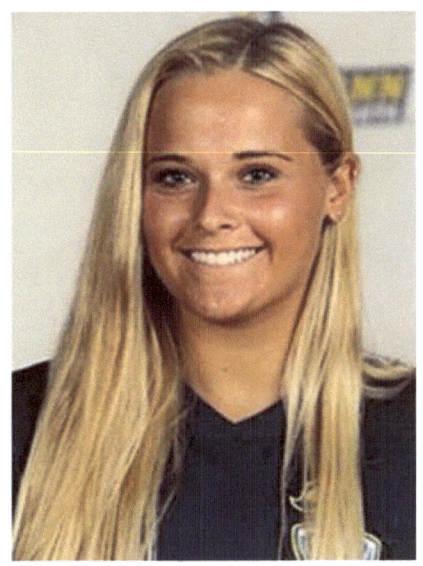

Meet Jennifer Collins

Jennifer writes…

"My name is Jennifer Collins and I am a sophomore college student at Neumann University in Aston, PA. I am also a communications major and a member of the women's soccer team at my university. I call Wildwood Crest, NJ home, where I live with my mother Jackie, father Mark, brother Daniel, and sister Joan. Growing up with a disabled sister has extremely impacted my life and I would love to share a piece of my story with the world."

Living With Hope

By Patrick Brigham

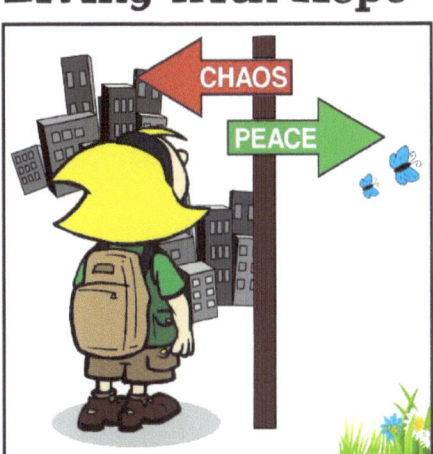

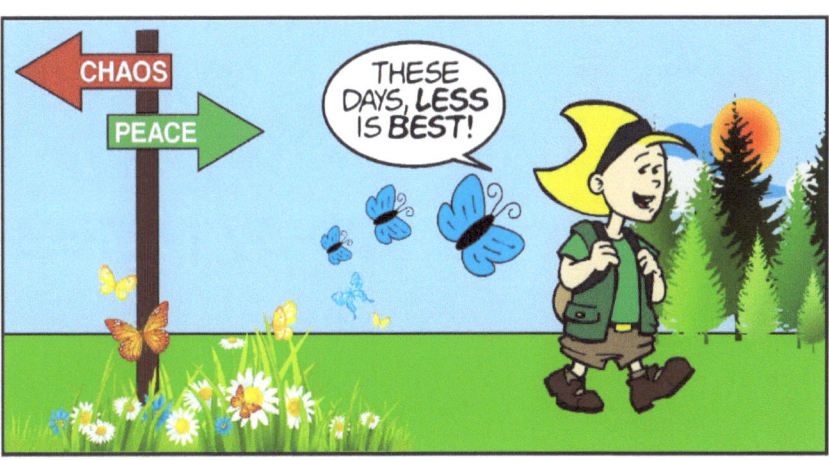

A Help Button Should Go Where You Go!

"Hello, this is MobileHelp. How may I assist you?"

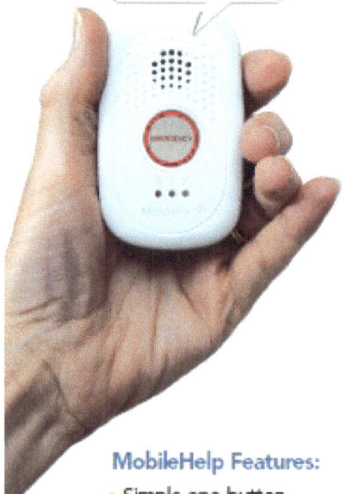

To be truly independent your personal emergency device needs to work on the go.

MobileHelp® allows you to summon emergency help 24 hours a day, 365 days a year by simply pressing your personal help button. Unlike traditional systems that only work inside your home, MobileHelp's medical alert system extends help beyond the home. Now you can participate in all your favorite activities such as gardening, taking walks, shopping and traveling all with the peace of mind of having a personal medical alert system with you. MobileHelp, the "on-the-go" help button, is powered by one of the nation's largest cellular networks, so there's virtually no limit to your help button's range.* With our GPS feature activated, we can send help to you, even when you can't talk or tell us where you are.

No landline? No Problem! While traditional medical alert systems require a landline, with MobileHelp's system, a landline is not necessary. Whether you are home or away from home, a simple press of your help button activates your system, providing the central station with your information and location. Our trained emergency operators will know who you are and where you are located.

If you're one of the millions of people that have waited for a medical alert service because it didn't fit your lifestyle, or settled for a traditional system even though it only worked in the home, then we welcome you to try MobileHelp. Experience peace of mind in the home or on the go.

MobileHelp Features:

- Simple one-button operation
- Affordable service
- Amplified 2-way voice communication
- 24/7/365 access to U.S. based operators
- GPS location detection
- Available Nationwide

As seen on:

Unlike 'stay-at-home' emergency systems MobileHelp protects you:		
Places where your Help Button will work	MobileHelp	Traditional Help Buttons
Home	✓	✓
On a Walk	✓	✗
On Vacation	✓	✗
At the Park	✓	✗
Shopping	✓	✗

Order Now & Receive a FREE Lockbox!

Place your door key in this box so that emergency personnel can get help to you even faster.

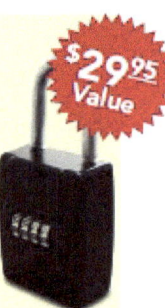

$29.95 Value

Optional Fall Button™

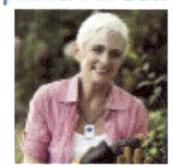

The automatic fall detect pendant that works **WHERE YOU GO!**

MobileHelp

1-800-371-2132

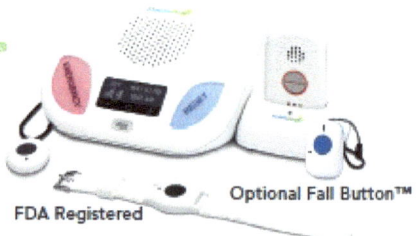

FDA Registered

Optional Fall Button™

 A+ BBB

*Service availability and access/coverage on the AT&T network is not available everywhere and at all times. Fall Button™ does not detect 100% of falls. If able, users should always push their help button when they need assistance. Current GPS location may not always be available in every situation. MobileHelp is a registered trademark and Fall Button is a trademark of MobileHelp. Patented technology. NBC, CBS News, The Early Show and The New York Times are registered trademarks. The use of the logos does not imply endorsement of MobileHelp from those organizations. MobileHelp is a FDA registered Medical Device Manufacturer.   MHP-006274E

Sharing is Better than Sulking

By Debra Gorman

Brain injury insists upon my constant attention and focus. I suffer but am grateful for the abilities I retain. Practicing gratitude is a big help to me emotionally. Suffering is part of our human condition, in one form or another. I truly believe that suffering has the potential to make us better and to soften us, as when leather is stretched and pummeled to render it soft, pliable and desirable.

I seldom whine about my circumstances and the toil that makes up every waking moment since my brain injury in 2011 and subsequent stroke. I plod along (literally) day by day being fairly independent. I try to care for others, although my caring looks nothing like it did pre-brain injury. The negative side of not whining is that those close to me may expect more from me than I can deliver. I think even my husband forgets how much I struggle at times, and more than anyone else he is a witness.

> "The negative side of not whining is that those close to me may expect more from me than I can deliver."

When John is home, mostly weekends, he does a lot of cleaning up after me. Due to my double vision and subsequent lack of depth perception, as well as only being able to safely use my non-dominant hand and arm, I make a lot of messes in the kitchen. John often rescues me by cleaning up after me. I appreciate that, but what I haven't enjoyed so much is the way he would often laugh at me, incredulous that I could be so sloppy. My husband has a great sense of humor and loves to laugh, qualities that attracted me to him in the first place. Many times, to demonstrate my own ability to see the humor in my foibles, I would join him in head-shaking and tittering. There truly is a humorous aspect to it all. Recently though, I fought tears as John cleaned up my oven spill.

Later, I confessed to him that his reaction hurt my feelings and I felt he failed to understand how much it pained me to work so hard only to achieve a shoddy result. I feel really bad when I dump sugar and flour on the kitchen floor or break dishes. Usually, he is at work and I manage to clean up after myself. When he has been home, I have felt shame.

Sometimes, I truly hurt myself. Right now, I am sporting a wound on the inside of my right wrist after sustaining burns from the oven a few days ago. I have many scars in the same area from oven burns. I have one hand to work with and it's my uncoordinated one. Sometimes the dishes or pots are too heavy for me to lift in or out of the oven one-handed. I have also cut myself countless times trying to chop vegetables or trim meat. Meal prep must then pause while I wait for the bleeding to subside. I can't even properly apply a Band-Aid—not a pleasant reality for a registered nurse. To his credit, John was apologetic and had no idea about my hurt feelings. I don't think he has made sport of me since.

Perhaps I have been extra sensitive since last Saturday when we took our three grandsons to the local botanical gardens. I had prepared a picnic lunch which we consumed after walking for what seemed like several miles. Since my brain injury, I not only fatigue quickly and profoundly, I have very poor balance and have the sensation that I'm carrying approximately one hundred pounds on my back, one hundred percent of the time when I'm standing or walking. It's a malfunction of the vestibular (or balance) system, originating in the brain. A former marathon runner, I am likely to stumble over the most minor change of grade in the terrain. When John is with me he offers his arm to hold on to, which is helpful because I may not notice stairs or a curb.

I love spending time with my grandsons, but I became overly exhausted that day and it took several days to recuperate. What is the take-away from this confession? This life isn't for sissies and maybe stoicism is overrated. It's acceptable to share our feelings and struggles with people who care; after all, our friends and loved ones cannot read our minds. Maybe suffering in silence is not the most noble of acts. How will they know if we don't communicate? Grief and pain of any kind has its own timetable. It should not be rushed. It will not be rushed. There is a way to share our struggles while being kind, non-accusatory and to ask for what we need. Sharing is better than sulking.

Meet Debra Gorman

Debra Gorman was fifty-six years old when she experienced her brain injuries. The first was a cavernous angioma, causing her brain to bleed, and four months later, a subdural hematoma. She later learned that she also had suffered a stroke during one of those events. She finds a creative outlet in writing. She is able to use a keyboard, tapping keys with her non-dominant forefinger and thumb. She enjoys writing for her children and grandchildren and has written articles that have been published for hospice. Currently, she writes for her blog, entitled Graceful Journey. debralynn48.wordpress.com.

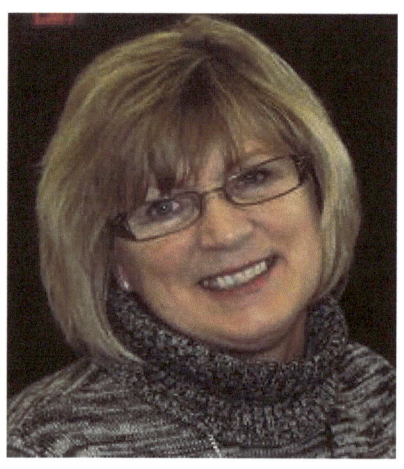

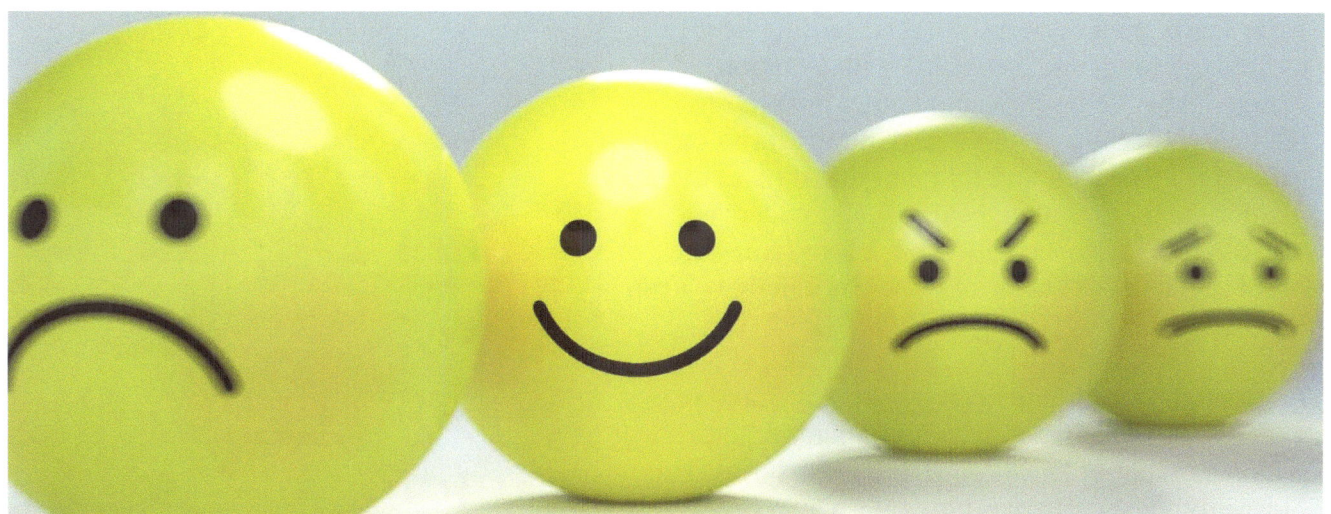

The Power of Positivity

By Rhonda Johnson

Brandon was a strong, athletic, handsome, and charismatic young man in his junior year of high school. He was very social and had many friends. I used to love watching his football games. Although he was smaller than most of the other kids, he was so fast he could dart in and out around everyone and carry the ball to touchdown time and time again!

But all of that changed when a car pulled out in front of my youngest son on his motorcycle just two days after his eighteenth birthday. Along with a compound fracture on his lower leg, shattered right hand, open book pelvic fracture, broken jaw on each side, punctured lung, broken rib, bruised heart, carotid arteries on each side of his neck, he also had a traumatic brain injury.

> "All of that changed when a car pulled out in front of my youngest son on his motorcycle just two days after his eighteenth birthday."

In the beginning, the focus was on fixing all of his broken parts. When we got through four surgeries in five days, a doctor discussed the scan showing the five places in his brain that were "injured" (damage is irreparable…but injuries are not!) They labeled it a "sheering" injury and said he "may" never wake up from his coma. I relied on the word "may" and thought "you don't know Brandon like I do – the stubborn warrior that he is!" I kept thinking that if he was going to die, he would have on the road. I know him – it's all or nothing!

After regrouping myself from this startling news, I cleared the room and had a chat with Brandon. Knowing that he worries about other people's feelings (especially mine), I gave him permission to pass on if he needed to. I told him that if he felt this was too much for him to beat, I would understand. A tear formed on each side of his eyes, so I knew he heard me. I said, "Then I'm in! If you can do it, I can do it too!"

From then on, I did my best to surround Brandon with positivity. No more negative doctor reports within ear-shot of Brandon. Happy hearts heal! His older brother, Jarrett, was home for winter break from college in Santa Cruz. We played his favorite music, had prayer circles around him, and read funny uplifting books. In quiet moments, I would lay my hands on him and beg God to take my energy and strength to heal my son. I would also whisper affirmations to him and remind him that I have his back. He could focus on healing and I'd take care of the rest.

Some people wanted to hear statistics asking, "What are his chances?" The idea of resigning to a statistic seemed ridiculous to me. Besides, anything physical that Brandon had ever done was always in the top 10%, up there with his brothers. Whatever numbers the neurologist rattled off sounded like excellent odds to my ears. While somewhere tucked away in a corner I knew there was a possibility he "may" never rally up, it wasn't where I chose to focus or expend energy. We had quite a mountain to climb, and I needed all my strength for that. Just for today, we are going to act "as if!"

After a month at Harborview, Brandon got sepsis poisoning from his feeding tube. All the progress made in a month seemed lost. It was as if he had finally gotten his nose above water, just to be kicked back down to the bottom of the pool. He was back in the ICU, back on a ventilator, and extremely ill. The sepsis seemed much worse than the wreck. He had to go through emergency surgery which was basically fileting his stomach open and flushing out his organs and body. He looked like a grape about to explode.

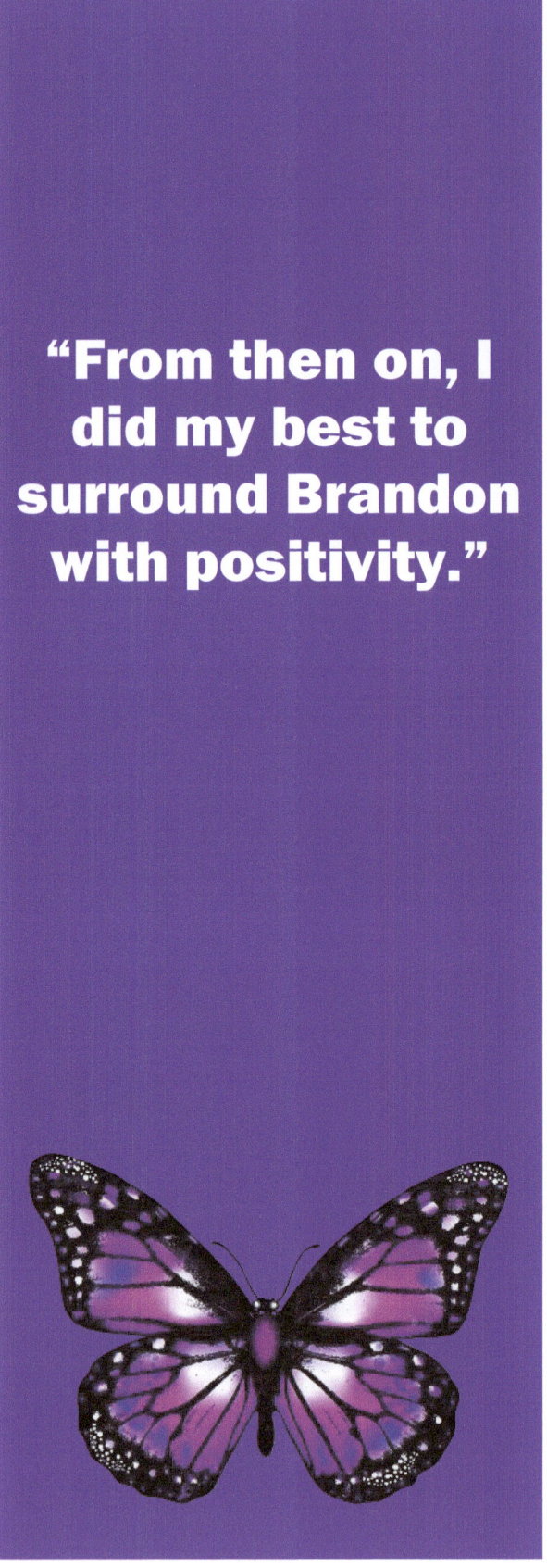

"From then on, I did my best to surround Brandon with positivity."

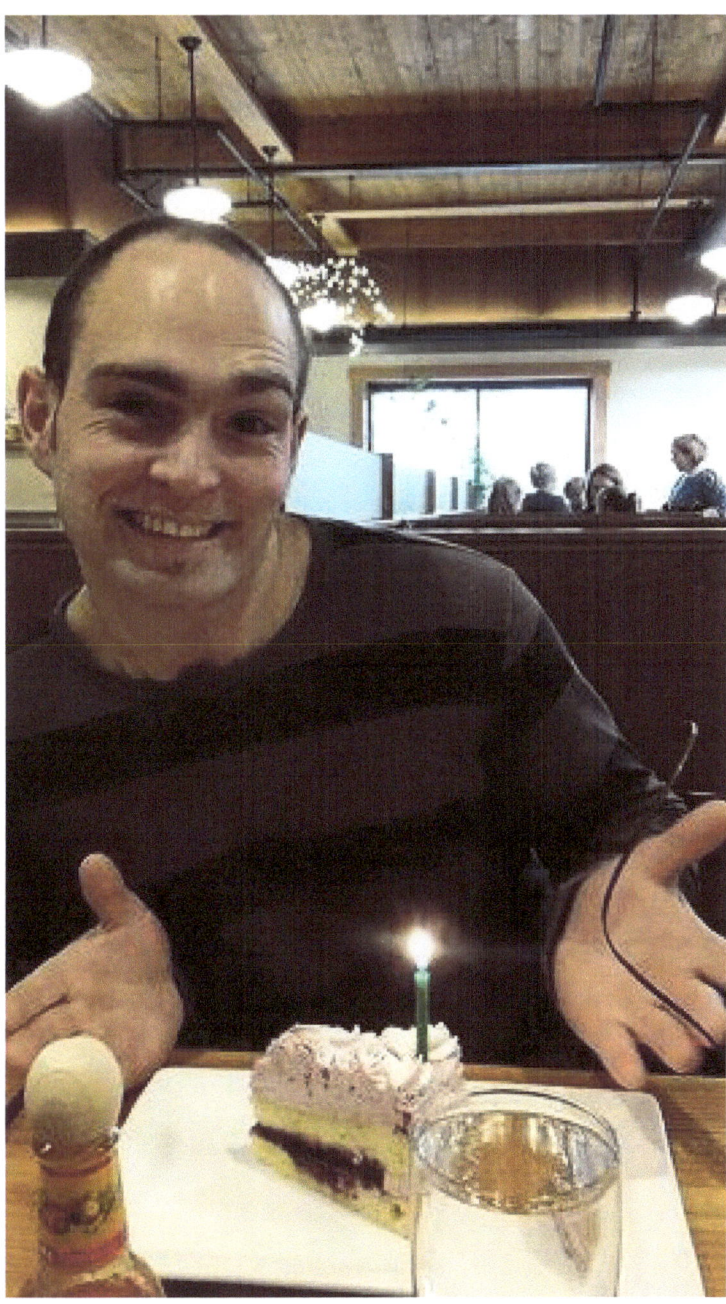

Brandon's Twenty-seventh Birthday

Even his face distorted while enduring so much physical pain. When his brother, Jarrett, saw him he backed up against the wall in the hallway and sank to his knees in tears. He asked, "How can you do this day after day?" It was a horrific ordeal and I truly didn't think he would make it since he had already been through so much. It was time. The Red Cross flew his oldest brother, a Marine in Afghanistan, home. It was touch and go for a few days, but he miraculously made it through the sepsis as well.

When it was finally time for discharge, I could not find the right care center for an eighteen-year-old young man who couldn't even push his call button (and after the sepsis incident I didn't want to risk it), so I found "Rehab Without Walls" and brought him home. At this point he was still unable to walk, talk or eat; he was still "storming" and he could not clear his own secretions. He had an open wound in his stomach from the sepsis surgery which needed to be packed with gauze and changed every twelve hours until it healed from the inside up.

My knowledge of Mother Nature and nutrition told me there's no way he could heal without whole foods abundant with live enzymes, so I started juicing for him. Just one apple perked him up like watering a wilted flower! I slowly added carrots, greens, vegetable soups and broth, probiotics, a raw multi-vitamin and mineral supplement and plenty of omega oils. Again, the room (now our living room) was filled with love, laughter and positivity.

The words, "I believe in you!" and "You can do this!" were repeated over and over. A chiropractor made twice weekly house calls for adjustments and laser therapy on his brain and open wound. I got him outside for fresh air whenever possible. As soon as funds were available (about a year after the accident), he did twenty-five rounds in a hyperbaric oxygen chamber.

Three years after his accident, Brandon still struggles with short-term memory loss, delusional thoughts (dreams and thoughts that mesh with reality) and paranoia. When someone meets him, they think he is drunk. He gets fatigued easily and often. However, Brandon is handsome, polite, charming, witty and funny. He can walk, talk, eat, and ride his bike. He is extremely active and walks, rides his bike, and works out at the gym every day. If you get an opportunity to run into Brandon and ask him how he is doing, he usually responds with, "Wonderful!" He is absolutely amazing and inspirational.

Words cannot describe how grateful I am for his strength. He still has a long way to go in his recovery, but when we look at how far he has climbed in three years it's truly amazing. Each month I see improvements. Some days are better than others but like I tell him, "Two steps forward and one back still gets you there!"

Meet Rhonda Johnson

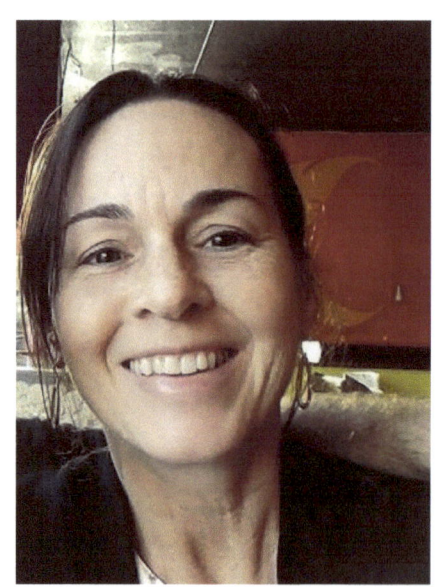

Rhonda calls the Pacific Northwest home. In the years since her son's traumatic brain injury, she has advocated on behalf of Brandon and other brain injury survivors. She is currently working on a book about her experiences and hopes that by sharing details of her own journey, others will be helped along the way.

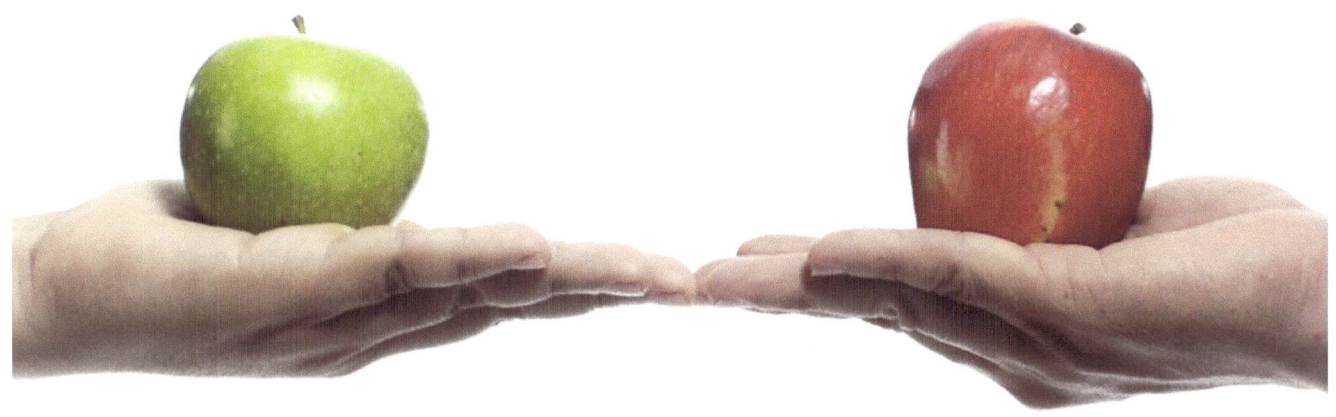

The Comparison Trap
By Norma Myers

We can all relate to being guilty of spinning around in the dizzying comparison trap. Whether it's love, family, career, financial, fashion, weight or cosmetic, somewhere along the line, we have compared ourselves to others. With the presence of social media, this trap has become even more intrusive.

From the moment we received the life-changing news of Aaron and Steven's car accident, the comparison trap began. Aaron didn't survive the accident that left Steven with a severe Traumatic Brain Injury (TBI). While the comparison trap from the loss of Aaron would set in later, it immediately bombarded us during Steven's recovery.

> "From the moment we received the life-changing news of Aaron and Steven's car accident, the comparison trap began."

Of all comparisons we thought we would face as parents, nothing prepared our ears to absorb the speech that began: don't compare your child's TBI progress to another survivor. A wonderful physician, who is now a friend, spoke those words to us. He then proceeded to inform us, "In a line-up of 10 TBI survivors, you would witness 10 different outcomes." *I did not want my son in a TBI line up or any part of the TBI community.*

All I wanted was to be able to turn back the calendar to August 13, 2012 and plan a totally different Sunday for our intact family of 4, a day close to home, together.

During Steven's roller-coaster recovery, we were reminded often, felt like hourly, that with the severity of Steven's injuries the recovery road was long, we should not get our hopes up. *Really?* Telling parents not to get their hopes up about their child's survival was the same as telling us not to take our next breath! Of course, we were going to hope, pray, and never give up. We admit, despite celebrating Steven's recovery, we did fall into the dismal comparison trap.

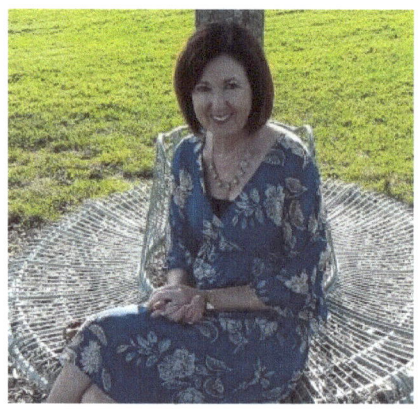

Meet Norma Myers

Norma and her husband Carlan spend much of their time supporting their son Steven as he continues on his road to recovery. Norma is an advocate for those recovering from traumatic brain injury.

Her written work has been featured on Brainline.org, a multi-media website that serves the brain injury community. Her family continues to heal.

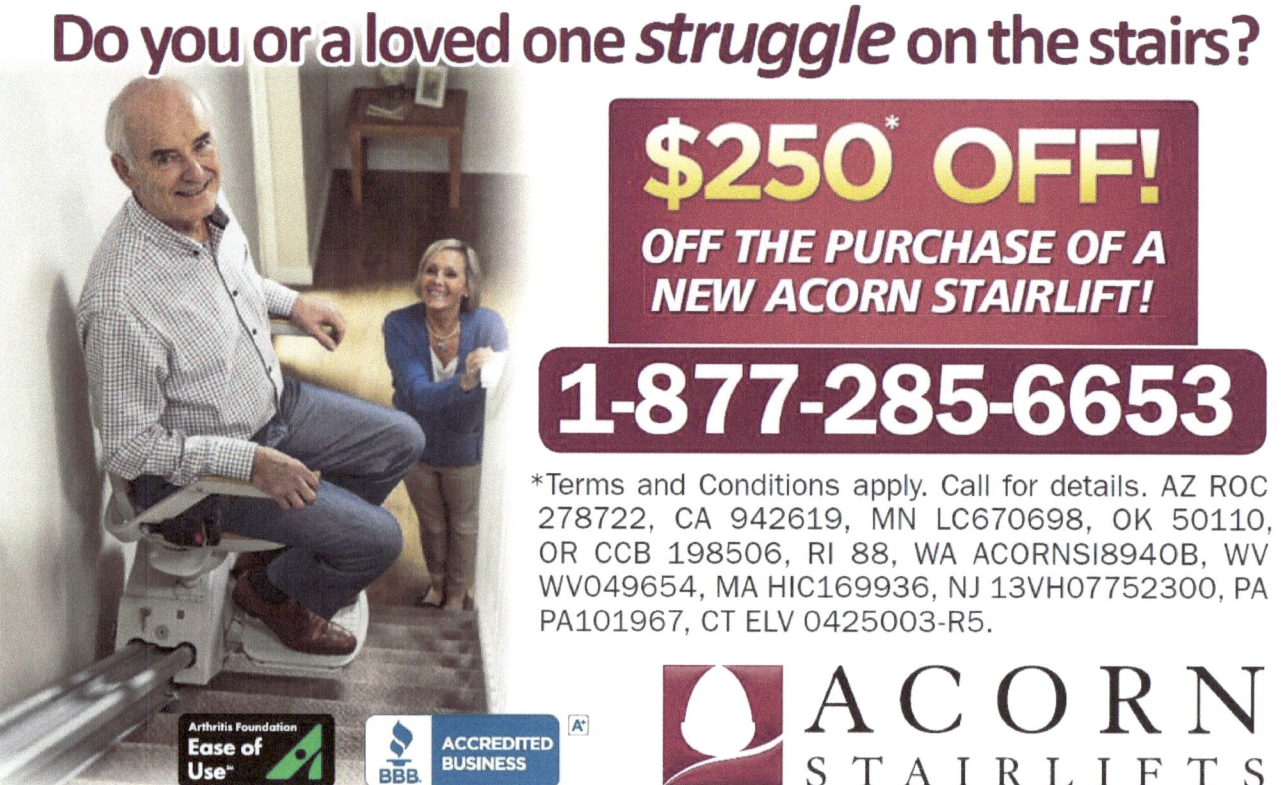

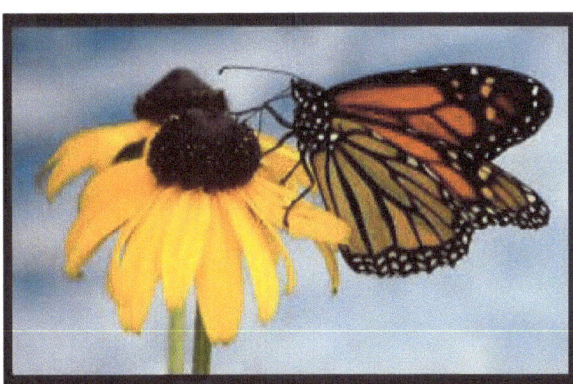
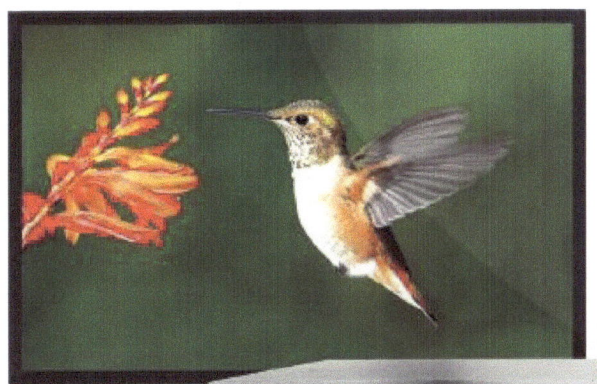
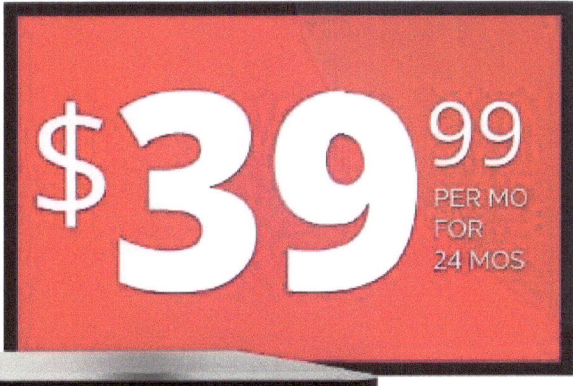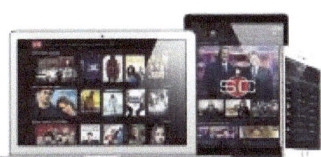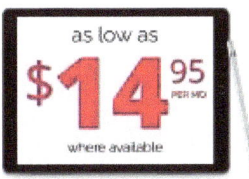

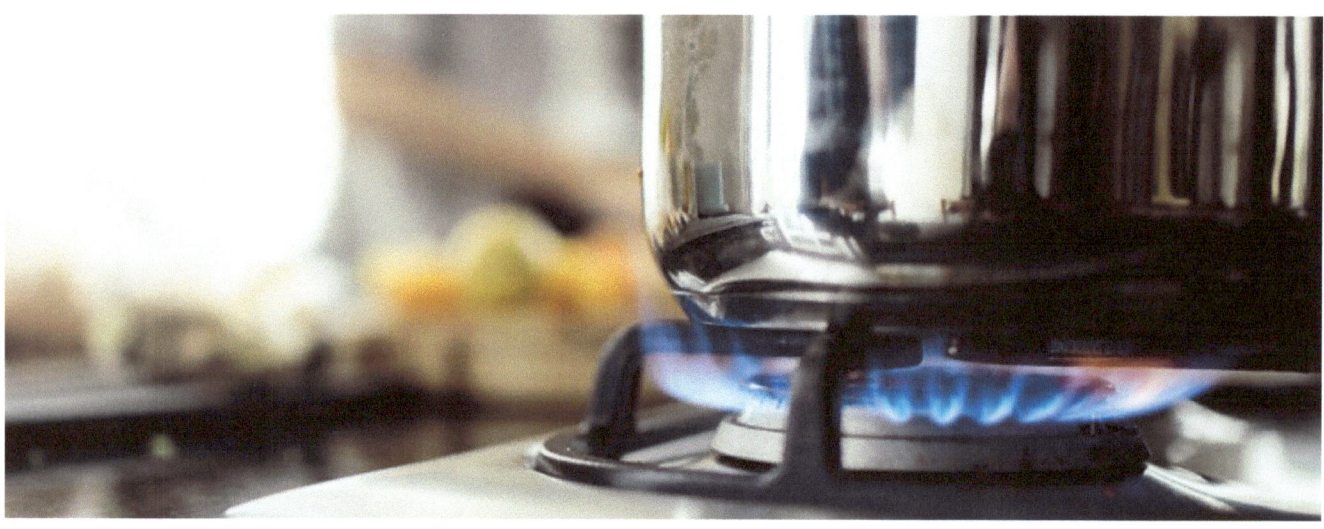

Forgetting the Burner is On

By Nicole Bingaman

Recently I planned to attend an evening yoga class. The class was on a Monday, a day I often take off of work to spend with Taylor, due to not having a caregiver. At some point in the afternoon I canceled the class because I felt entirely drained. The day started with tremendous emotional turbulence. Thankfully, I was able to contain the gush of caregiver anxiety I was experiencing. However, containing the emotions depleted my reserves. By 2:30 p.m. I was exhausted. And both Taylor and I settled in for a nap.

The initial hours of the morning were hard. I woke up with unexpected energy, knowing I had to clean. My house and especially the bathrooms were in dire need of attention. The dining room floor looked as if it hadn't been vacuumed in weeks, and my to-do list was growing. However, Taylor had his own list of things that must be done. He was following me around the house, chomping at the bit, and his anxiousness added to my unease.

I decided to choose three things that couldn't wait, and then move on with our day. I felt like I was in a pressure cooker. It was as if some angry drill sergeant was screaming in my head, "Get it done. NOW!" The demands of life and caregiving had caught up, and they were messing with mind and body. My heart was pounding, my brain was unsettled.

Caregiving is challenging. I shy away from sharing the truth of how fatigued I feel, as I know some of you do. I fear people will think I am constantly hosting a pity party. Full-time, live-in caregivers understand being tired in a way others don't. This is not a pity party we are hosting, it is an *"I am so exhausted I can't see straight party!"*

People ask why Taylor can't be left alone. The answer is complex. I will scratch the surface. Taylor has major deficits with his executive functioning skills. He doesn't notice certain things, like huge weights crashing to the ground if not properly secured when lifting, or a car coming towards him on the road. We practiced that exercise once- using the crosswalk while I observed from afar. Um, not pretty. His mind fails to bear witness and register the smaller things.

This might be described as the "forgetting the burner is on while the pan scorches syndrome." Taylor's brain injury means he can't always connect the dots. He lacks insight about actions and their consequences. His caregiving needs are not just about his seizure disorder. His needs are about his decision-making skills, large and small. And more, much more.

I was super tensed up. And it showed. I explained to Taylor that I was not mad at him, but I was upset and overwhelmed. One of the gifts of my relationship with Taylor is that we communicate in a very real way. This is powerful.

> **"One of the gifts of my relationship with Taylor is that we communicate in a very real way. This is powerful."**

Later, I felt horrible about how the morning went. Not a pretty series of minutes for me. Picture an angry, overwhelmed, stressed out, caregiver meltdown. I had it. The outward expression wasn't too dramatic, but the inward turmoil was amped up in a way that rattled me.

Three nights later I made it to my yoga class. I entered the studio with such intense gratitude for the space I could offer myself over the next hour.

As the class began, we were led to a mantra called Ho'oponopono, an ancient Hawaiian prayer. This mantra is a reflection of forgiveness of yourself or someone else. And goes like this:

Please forgive me.
I am so sorry.
I love you.
Thank you.

Throughout the practice, I whispered those words to Taylor and myself as I moved within my own body, I felt peace. From within I spoke, full of love and sincerity.
Please forgive me, Taylor.
I am sorry for your injury and the tremendous pain it has caused you.
I love you my son. So very much.
Thank you for the love you've offered me.
Then to myself.
Please forgive me.

I am sorry this continues to be difficult and painful.
I love you, Nicole. So much.
Thank you for being present and showing up, every single day.

My eyes were closed as I moved through parts of the class. At some point, I returned to a memory of Taylor. It was summertime. He must have been 19 or twenty. We were at the Yorktown beach. Taylor was smiling at me and the sun was shining behind him. He was so gorgeous, glowing from the inside out. I took a deep breath and said, "I miss you." as tears fell down my face.

Suddenly, I realized the missing is really what the angst was about. The missing of what was...the dreams, the plans, and the struggles that have replaced them. The struggles I seldom share, the wounds that seem to be picked again and again. And the fact that I didn't expect my life or Taylor's to ever look like this. We live in a world I never once imagined or anticipated. And sometimes I still feel ill-prepared for.

The lack of understanding of what it means to live with ambiguous grief and the isolation it often presents hurts me.

I see this image of my son, and I can't help but miss the person I see. But this person is still here. There is a voice saying, "Don't share your grief." The voice reminds me I don't want to be judged or called out (even silently) for my feelings. Missing a person who is still here. What is that? That is life with my son's brain injury. That is ambiguous grief.

At the end of the practice I promised myself to practice courage by sharing hard truth and loving myself through it. I can't say this enough...Caregivers, I see you. You are not alone. You are dearly loved. You matter. You are enough. And so am I.

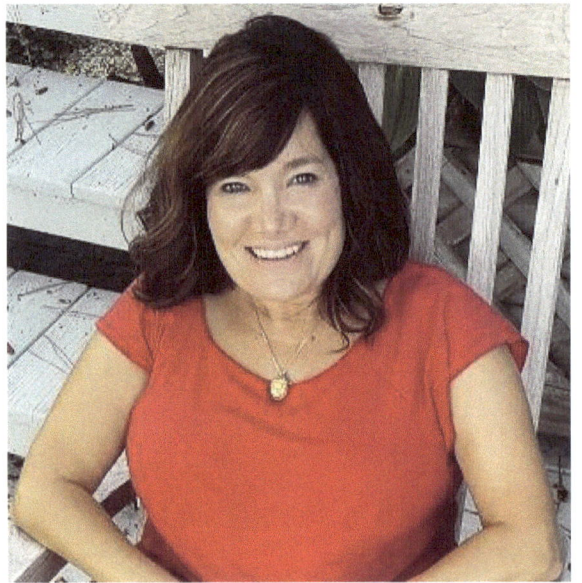

Meet Nicole Bingaman

Nicole writes…

My name is Nicole Bingaman. I became a student in the classroom of traumatic brain injury over five years ago. Since that time, I have learned that love does win, but that love is also made up of incredibly tough moments. By giving myself permission to tell the truth, I hope that there can be healing for others who are walking this same road

News & Views

If you want to get a real feeling for the tenacity of the human spirit, take a moment to look around the brain injury community. While our community is one that experiences many challenges, it is also defined by the overcoming of seemingly insurmountable obstacles.

This issue of HOPE Magazine has more stories by family members of brain injury survivors than any prior issue. Now in our ninth year as a survivor family, we have personally experienced many of the life challenges that you've just read about.

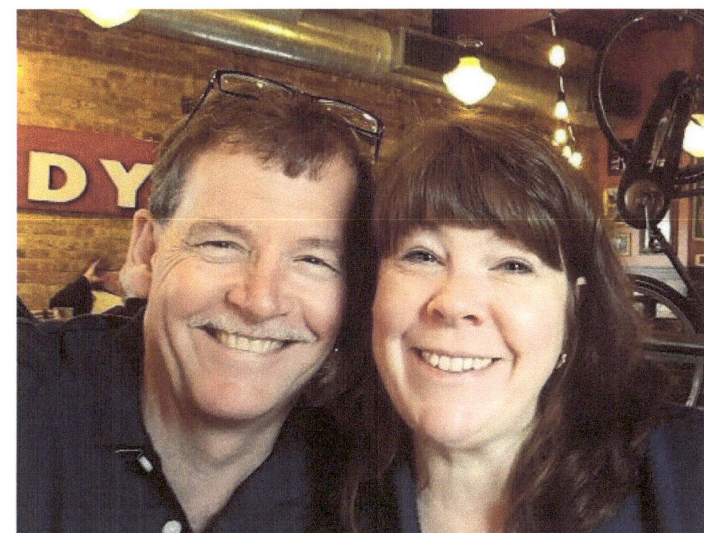

But we found our way.

Brain injury recovery does indeed have a start date, a date often defined by trauma, accident, or unforeseeable circumstance. But happily, there is no end-date on recovery. Contrary to what was taught a few short years ago, recovery does not end after a year, in fact, as we can attest to, recovery is ongoing.

A heartfelt thank you to this month's contributors. Without those brave souls willing to be open and transparent about their struggles, others who share the same fate would do so alone, never really knowing that others truly do understand.

Peace.

~David and Sarah

www.ingramcontent.com/pod-product-compliance
Lightning Source LLC
Chambersburg PA
CBHW060806290526
45792CB00005BA/1544